BIBLE CURE®

FOR

THYROID
DISORDERS

Don Colbert, M.D.

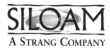

A Strang Company

THE BIBLE CURE FOR THYROID DISORDERS
by Don Colbert, M.D.
Published by Siloam
A Strang Company
600 Rinehart Road
Lake Mary, Florida 32746
www.siloam.com

by the Lockman Foundation. Used by permission.
(www.Lockman.org)

Scripture quotations marked NIV are from the Holy
Bible, New International Version. Copyright © 1973,
1978, 1984, International Bible Society. Used by
permission.

Library of Congress Catalog Card Number:
2003112466
International Standard Book Number: 1-59185-281-1

This book is not intended to provide medical advice
or to take the place of medical advice and treatment
from your personal physician. Readers are advised
to consult their own doctors or other qualified
health professionals regarding the treatment of their
medical problems. Neither the publisher nor the
author takes any responsibility for any possible con-
sequences from any treatment, action or application
of medicine, supplement, herb or preparation to any
person reading or following the information in this
book. If readers are taking prescription medications,
they should consult with their physicians and not
take themselves off of medicines to start supplemen-
tation without the proper supervision of a physician.

04 05 06 07 08 — 9 8 7 6 5 4 3 2 1
Printed in the United States of America

Do You Have a Hidden Problem?

Feeling really tired lately? Perhaps you've gained weight or just can't seem to lose it no matter how hard you try. Are you cold all the time? Is your skin dryer than usual, or have you noticed that you seem extra thirsty or just achy? Maybe you've been kind of down, forgetful, constipated or unusually irritable. If any of these sound like you, you may be a part of a hidden epidemic: *hypothyroidism or low-thyroid function.*

If so, it's no accident that you've picked up this Bible Cure book. For God's Word declares that He works to bring hidden things to light. Luke 12:2 says, "But there is nothing covered up that will not be revealed, and hidden that will not be known" (NAS).

It's estimated that more than 13 million American women have some kind of thyroid dysfunction, and many of them do not know it. Men have it, too.[1]

Thyroid disorders hide in the darkness of our ignorance, far from view, which allows them to wreak havoc with our health and peace of mind. They are one of the most underdiagnosed problems today, and professionals easily miss many of their symptoms. In fact, experts estimate that more than half of those with low-grade hypothyroidism remain undiagnosed. Researchers say about 10 percent of younger women and 20 percent of women over fifty regularly experience mild thyroid problems that impact their weight, attitude and overall health.[2] As we will see, milder cases of thyroid disorder often do not show up in standard medical tests, yet they still create distressing symptoms.

Sadly, for the millions suffering from a thyroid disorder of which they are entirely unaware, the Bible says in Hosea 4:6, "My people are destroyed for lack of knowledge" (NAS). These individuals could be unknowingly harming their bodies by not eating the right foods or taking the right supplements or medications.

Nevertheless, I have good news for you. God wants you well and happy, and He is at work to bring hidden problems to light in order to heal them for you. In fact, He has wonderful plans for your life! He has a purpose for you—a special task on this earth only you can fulfill. The Bible clearly declares that God wishes above all things that you prosper and be in health, even as your soul prospers (3 John 2). God's wonderful plan for your life includes terrific, vibrant health.

Unfortunately, there is a devil who would like nothing more than to see you unable to fulfill your destiny. Jesus promised to give us life and life more abundantly. He also said that the purpose of the devil is to kill, steal and destroy (John 10:10). Your adversary will use every trick in the book to keep you down and defeated—and that includes bringing hidden sickness and disease upon your body. But God has revealed the wisdom we need through the field of medicine, natural remedies He has placed on this earth and, most powerfully, His mighty Word and healing power.

Spiritual Roots of Disease

As a Christian medical doctor, I have studied and prayed about the causes of disease for many years. Increasingly, I have discovered that many diseases have strong spiritual roots. God is interested in the health of the entire person—body, mind and spirit. Although traditional medicine often sees these facets of our being as separate, in truth they are not. A vital link exists between the spirit, soul and body. That's why this Bible Cure is strategically designed to bring God's healing power to your heart, mind and spirit through the power of faith and God's wonderful Word.

No matter what the cause is of your thyroid condition, with His help and with the truths you will learn from this book, you *will* overcome. This Bible Cure book is filled with hope and encouragement for understanding how to keep your body fit and in a healthy balance. In it you will

uncover God's divine plan of health for body, soul and spirit through modern medicine, good nutrition and the medicinal power of Scripture and prayer.

You will find key Scripture passages throughout this book that will help you focus on the power of God. These divine promises will empower your prayers and redirect your thoughts to line up with God's plan of divine health for you—a plan that includes victory over whatever thyroid condition may be afflicting you.

This Bible Cure book will give you a strategic plan for divine health as discussed in the following chapters:

If you are suffering from a thyroid disorder, take fresh confidence in the knowledge that God is real. He is alive, and He loves you more than you could ever imagine. You *will* enjoy complete restoration of your health—body, mind and spirit.

It is my prayer that these powerful godly insights will bring health, wholeness and spiritual refreshing to you. May they deepen your fellowship with God and strengthen your ability to worship and serve Him, fulfilling your divine purpose on the earth.

—DON COLBERT, M.D.

A BIBLE CURE PRAYER
FOR YOU

Heavenly Father, I pray that You will help apply the truths from this book as I trust You to help me with my thyroid disorders. Let Your wisdom guide me as I allow Your healing power to come to my body, mind and spirit through the power of faith and Your Word. In Jesus' name, amen.

Chapter 1

A Lamp of Understanding

The presence of God in your life is a constantly burning flame of wisdom, power, knowledge, peace and help. If you let Him, He will light a pathway to total restoration and radiant refreshing. In fact, the Bible says, "Your word is a lamp for my feet and a light for my path" (Ps. 119:105).

The first step along your pathway is wisdom and understanding. "Happy is the person who finds wisdom and gains understanding....Wisdom is a tree of life to those who embrace her" (Prov. 3:13, 18). You may wonder, *How do I get this wisdom?* It's really not complicated. The Bible says simply go out and get it.

Therefore, let's begin this Bible Cure by taking the first step: gaining a good understanding of the thyroid and its disorders. In this chapter you will discover whether you may have a thyroid disorder and what it means if you do.

1

Your Thyroid

Until a problem occurs, most people never consider their thyroid gland or how important it is to the health of their bodies. The thyroid actually has a shape similar to a butterfly, with two lobes that extend like wings. They stretch across the front of the lower part of your neck, straddling your windpipe between your breastbone and Adam's apple.

What You Should Know

The main purpose of the thyroid gland is to produce and release two hormones that are vitally important to your body: T3 (or triiodothyronine) and T4 (or thyroxine).

The signal for thyroid hormone production actually begins in the brain. The part of the brain called the *hypothalamus* produces a hormone called TRH (thyrotropin-releasing hormone). This hormone is sent to the pituitary gland beneath the hypothalamus, which triggers it to release TSH (thyroid-stimulating hormone). The TSH leaves the pituitary gland and travels in the bloodstream to the thyroid, eventually causing the production and release of the thyroid hormones T3 and T4.

The delicate balance of these hormones makes a great difference to your health. When your body receives too little of these hormones, you will experience *hypothyroidism*, a disease process caused by an *underactive* thyroid gland. Hormones dramatically affect many of the body's systems and functions. That's why low levels of these vital hormones can create a wide range of problems; they impact nearly everything your body tries to do. That includes breaking down fat, regulating menstrual periods and controlling body temperature. With an underactive thyroid,

> *Praise the LORD, I tell myself, and never forget the good things he does for me. He forgives all my sins and heals all my diseases.*
> —PSALM 103:2–3

you might experience a weight gain that seems impossible to lose no matter how hard you try.

Hyperthyroidism, just the opposite condition, is caused by an *overactive* thyroid gland. In other words, your body gets too much of these vital hormones, causing you to lose weight, sweat a lot, feel hot when others are comfortable and have a rapid heart rate. Nevertheless, it's still possible to have one of these conditions and experience absolutely no symptoms at all, which is part of the hidden nature of this problem.

Let's examine the symptoms of thyroid disorder a little more closely to help you determine whether or not some of your symptoms are being caused by thyroid hormone imbalance.

When Your Body Attacks Itself

In the United States as well as in Europe, the primary cause of hypothyroidism is an autoimmune thyroid disease called Hashimoto's thyroiditis. Here your immune system begins attacking your own thyroid gland as if it were a threatening invader. Over time, the thyroid becomes damaged, eventually resulting in hypothyroidism.

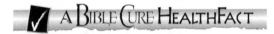

✔ A BIBLE CURE HEALTHFACT

Do You Have Symptoms?

Answer the following questions to determine if you could have symptoms of an underactive thyroid gland:

- ❑ Do you have unexplained fatigue?
- ❑ Are you weak?
- ❑ Are you lethargic?
- ❑ Are you experiencing unwanted weight gain?
- ❑ Do you have dry skin? Flaky skin?

- ❑ Are you experiencing hair loss?
- ❑ Are you more irritable lately?
- ❑ Are you constipated?
- ❑ Are your hands and feet cold?
- ❑ Are you depressed?
- ❑ Do you have problems concentrating?
- ❑ Are you having irregular menstrual cycles?
- ❑ Do you forget people's names easily?
- ❑ Do you have puffiness and swelling around the eyes, face, feet or hands?
- ❑ Has your voice become hoarse?
- ❑ Are you unable to lose weight with proper diet and exercise?
- ❑ Do you have a history of miscarriages?

HEALTHFACT HEALTHFACT HEALTHFACT HEALTHFACT HEALTHFACT HEALTHFACT HEALTHFACT

In the quiz above, no single question points to a thyroid disorder, but if you answered *yes* to several of these questions, it is quite possible that you may be suffering from a thyroid imbalance. I strongly recommend that you have your thyroid gland checked by a medical professional who can draw a blood test for TSH and free T4 levels. Also, take this questionnaire to your doctor to more thoroughly discuss your symptoms with him.

Some of the more common symptoms of hypothyroidism are listed in the previous Bible Cure Health Fact, but one unexpected symptom is the thinning of the hair, especially if the hair becomes more brittle and breaks easily, or if you lose the hair in the outer third of your eyebrows.

Many individuals with hypothyroidism experience some degree of depression. A decreased sex drive, infertility, problems achieving pregnancy, menstrual cycle irregularities and an increased risk of miscarriage are also fairly common and unfortunate characteristics of hypothyroidism.

Other symptoms include irritability, muscle weakness, swelling in the neck, brittle nails, elevated cholesterol levels and achy joints. Yet, we've seen that some people have no symptoms at all, which is why it's so important for you to get tested.

Hide and Seek

OK, you say you've been to the doctor and had your thyroid tested, and the results came back as normal. Still you continue to experience a number of symptoms associated with thyroid problems. Before you decide that you have become a hypochondriac, consider this: thyroid levels can fluctuate, and thyroid disease can turn itself on and off. It works a little like the appliance that you finally take to the repair shop, only to find that when the repairman plugs it in it works just fine.

Just because you've received a clean bill of health following a blood test does not mean you're home free. You may still have a slight thyroid condition that is not showing up in the blood tests, or your hormone levels may simply be a little off balance temporarily. The results are the same: you

> *But he was wounded and crushed for our sins. He was beaten that we might have peace. He was whipped, and we were healed!*
> —ISAIAH 53:5

feel tired, gain weight or experience any of the many other symptoms of thyroid dysfunction.

More experts are realizing that slight fluctuations in thyroid hormones—problems that often do not show up in medical tests—are creating the same distressing symptoms for millions of people.

Women who are experiencing the normal hormonal fluctuations that accompany menopause and peri- or premenopause may experience low thyroid. Low thyroid is the suspected culprit in a host of underlying symptoms of menopause that often go undiagnosed. In fact, by age fifty, one in every twelve women has a significant degree of hypothyroidism. By age sixty, it is one woman out of every six.[1]

A BIBLE CURE HEALTH TIP

Get a Checkup!

The American Thyroid Association recommends that serum TSH screening be instituted at age thirty-five in both men and women and be repeated every five years.[2]

Getting an Accurate Diagnosis

During medical school and throughout my residency, I began to notice that some individuals who had normal TSH levels continued to experience many symptoms of low thyroid. The TSH test is the main blood test to diagnose and manage hypothyroidism.

A normal TSH is considered to be in the range of 0.5 to 5 microunits per milliliter. Yet, today the

American Association of Clinical Endocrinologists (AACE) now says that a TSH level between 3.0 and 5.0 microunits per milliliter should be considered representative of hypothyroidism. Despite this official change, many doctors have patients whose TSH levels are between 3 and 5 and who are displaying symptoms of hypothyroidism, yet they continue to dismiss the diagnosis of thyroid disease. The higher the TSH test, the more hypothyroid you are.

Screen Yourself to Be Sure

If you suspect your thyroid may be acting up, here's a simple test you can give yourself at home to let you know whether you may have a sluggish thyroid condition.

A BIBLE CURE HEALTH TIP

Track Your Basal Body Temperature

Some doctors believe that blood tests may not be sensitive enough to detect milder forms of hypothyroidism. This test is easy and is a great indicator of a milder or intermittent form of thyroid dysfunction. I suggest you try it even if you're in doubt. Simply follow these steps:

1. Place a thermometer next to your night stand, but shake it down first to be sure it registers below 95 degrees Fahrenheit. Be sure you can reach it easily without getting out of bed.

2. The following morning before you rise, take your temperature by placing the thermometer under your armpit for ten minutes. Remain as still as possible.

3. Record your temperature reading for at least three consecutive days.

Women should do this during the first two weeks of their menstrual cycle to get an accurate reading. The first day of the menstrual period is the first day of the menstrual cycle.

Normal basal body temperatures fall between 97.4 and 98.2 degrees Fahrenheit. If your reading is consistently below 97.4, you could be hypothyroid.

Many individuals have consistently low basal body temperatures and experience many of the symptoms of hypothyroidism. Yet their thyroid blood tests are normal. For these individuals I recommend further blood tests, including thyroid autoantibodies.

The Other Extreme: Hyperthyroidism

We have seen what happens when the body doesn't get enough thyroid hormone, but you may be wondering what happens if it gets too much. This thyroid disease is called *hyperthyroidism*. It is far less common, affecting about 2 million Americans, compared to the 11 million suffering with an underactive thyroid.

Hyperthyroidism works much the opposite of hypothyroidism. Where hypothyroidism seems to slow down the body's metabolism, hyperthyroidism revs it up. A thyroid on high throttle can cause very distressing symptoms. Take the test below to see if you may be experiencing hyperthyroidism.

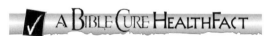

Symptoms of Hyperthyroidism

Answer the following questions to determine if you could have symptoms of an overactive thyroid gland:

❑ Do you have a rapid or irregular heartbeat?

❑ Do you feel nervous much of the time?

❑ Are you more irritable?

- ❏ Do your hands shake with tremors?
- ❏ Are you always hungry?
- ❏ Have you lost weight?
- ❏ Do you have a wide-eyed stare?
- ❏ Have you experienced more diarrhea?
- ❏ Do you have menstrual periods with scant bleeding?
- ❏ Are you infertile?
- ❏ Do you sweat a lot when others seem to be comfortable?
- ❏ Are you intolerant to heat?
- ❏ Do you tire quickly?
- ❏ Are your muscles weak?
- ❏ Are you having trouble sleeping?
- ❏ Are you experiencing mood swings?
- ❏ Are you experiencing shortness of breath?
- ❏ Is your hair fine and straight?
- ❏ Is it sometimes difficult to catch your breath?

Because thyroid disorder can hide from even the best medical examiners, no single symptom points to it. But if you answered *yes* to several of these symptoms, please get examined by your medical doctor or endocrinologist for hyperthyroidism. Remember that your thyroid helps your body to perform many vital functions, so never take a possible problem lightly.

What You Need to Know

Women are ten times more likely than men to develop hyperthyroidism.[3] The most common cause of hyperthyroidism is Graves' disease, an autoimmune disorder that may cause the thyroid gland to enlarge, usually forming what is known as a goiter. Other causes include an inflammation of the thyroid triggered by a viral infection or childbirth, or the formation of localized lumps or nodules in the gland itself that can cause it to produce too much thyroid hormone. Eating too much iodine may create the same effect; benign and malignant tumors can, too.

Dr. Robert Graves was a nineteenth-century Irish physician who first recognized this condition and consequently named it after himself. Graves' disease is caused when the body's immune system attacks the thyroid gland, especially the TSH receptors. Even after these receptors have been destroyed, the thyroid gland continues to release hormones into the bloodstream, flooding the body with excessive hormones, much like an engaged accelerator that is stuck in a car.

Graves' disease usually affects women between the ages of twenty and forty. Approximately 1 percent of the general population has Graves' disease.[4]

Signs and Symptoms

The most common symptoms of Graves' disease include a rapid pulse and heart palpitations. A person afflicted with this disease may even develop an arrhythmia of the heart, or atrial fibrillation, and it may cause heart failure in older patients.

Other symptoms are multiple and varied. Usually the thyroid gland is enlarged and firm. There is often a loss of muscle mass, which may cause extreme weakness.

Aside from the more common syptoms like those listed earier in the Health Fact, another symptom is weight loss, especially loss of muscle mass. Thyroid eye disease, or *exophthalmus*, is commonly associated with Graves' disease. Those with this problem seem to have bulging, watery eyes due to eyelid retraction in which the upper eyelid is pulled back, exposing more of the white of the eyes. About half of those with Graves' disease suffer from thyroid eye disease. However, the condition usually is mild and doesn't progress once the hyperthyroidism is controlled.

A final symptom of Graves' disease is a thyroid skin disease called *pretibial myxedema*. It is much less common than thyroid eye disease and only becomes severe in about 1 percent of Graves' disease sufferers. Thyroid skin disease looks like a thickening of the skin, usually in the front of the lower leg, which becomes raised and pink.

About 10 to 15 percent of those with Graves' disease have thyroid nodules, or small lumps in the thyroid. Let's take a look.

> *Pay attention, my child, to what I say. Listen carefully. Don't lose sight of my words. Let them penetrate deep within your heart, for they bring life and radiant health to anyone who discovers their meaning.*
> —PROVERBS 4:20–22

Thyroid Nodules

While they can be disturbing to think about at first, nodules of the thyroid gland are fairly common. In fact, about one in every fifteen women and one in every sixty men have a thyroid nodule—and they may not even know it![5]

A nodule is simply a small lump on the thyroid gland. It can be the size of a small pea to the size of a ping-pong ball or even larger. The good news is that the majority of thyroid nodules—in fact, over 90 percent—are benign. And even if nodules do become cancerous, they are curable about 90 percent of the time.

If you have a thyroid nodule, ask your doctor to perform thyroid function tests. Get a "free T4" and a TSH test, and also have a fine needle aspiration biopsy. ("Free T4" is the actual name of the blood test.) Some doctors perform thyroid scans as well as thyroid ultrasound studies to check a thyroid nodule, but a fine needle biopsy is a more specific procedure that may allow you to skip the thyroid scan and the ultrasound.

Goiters

Approximately 200 million people worldwide suffer from goiters, a disturbing condition that appears as a swelling in the front of the neck.[6] A goiter is simply a swelling of the thyroid gland—a structural disorder that may be caused by Graves' or Hashimoto's disease. Another type of goiter that may occur in postmenopausal women is a multinodular goiter. Here, instead of the thyroid developing one lump, it develops multiple nodules, which are usually benign.

Causes of goiters

Goiters can be due to a number of factors: iodine insufficiency, hyperthyroidism, hypothyroidism and multinodular goiters. Most of the time, a goiter indicates that the thyroid gland is straining to produce enough hormones. However, it could also mean you are not getting enough iodine in your diet.

"Goiter Belts" was a term used to refer to areas of the country in which people often did not have adequate amounts of iodine in their diets—resulting in goiters. The Great Lakes region was once considered a goiter belt. Fortunately, goiters caused by iodine deficiency have all but been eliminated in the United States due to the development of iodized salt.

A Wise Creator

The psalmist said, "Bless the LORD, O my soul, and forget none of His benefits; who pardons all your iniquities; who heals all your diseases; who redeems your life from the pit; who crowns you with lovingkindness and compassion; who satisfies your years with good things, so that your youth is renewed like the eagle" (Ps. 103: 2–5, NAS). This passage holds a promise that God intends to heal you of every disease—and that includes thyroid disease. He will crown you with His wonderful love and fill your years with good things.

What a wonderful promise from a wise and loving Creator. Best yet, it is not just *a* promise; it is *your* promise. Why not bow your head for a minute and thank Him for His love and healing power in your life.

A BIBLE CURE PRAYER
FOR YOU

Heavenly Father, I praise You because I am fearfully and wonderfully made. I ask that You touch my thyroid gland right now and cause it to begin to function normally. I pray that You give my doctors the wisdom to understand the root cause of this thyroid disorder and to target the most effective treatment. Please restore my body from the top of my head to the soles of my feet so that I can carry out my divine purpose in the world. In Jesus' name, amen.

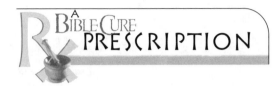

RX A BIBLE CURE PRESCRIPTION

Write a prayer concerning your current physical and emotional condition. Close it by thanking God for His healing touch.

_____

_____

_____

_____

_____

_____

_____

_____

_____

_____

_____

_____

Chapter 2

Full of Light—Lifestyle Factors

Glowing health throughout your body is a
shining light. The Bible suggests that your
physical well-being is directly linked to how
clearly you see God's light of truth and wisdom.
Luke 11:34 says, "Your eye is a lamp for your
body. A pure eye lets sunshine into your soul. But
an evil eye shuts out the light and plunges you
into darkness." In other words, seeing things in
the light of God's truth shines a radiant beacon of
good health and healing power throughout your
body.

In God's healing light, no sickness, disease or
affliction can hide. It's my prayer that your body
might be full of light, with God's wisdom and truth
bringing every system into perfect divine health.
That is God's very best for you—body, mind and
spirit.

Together let's shine the light of truth upon

hidden lifestyle factors that may be at the root of your thyroid problems.

Will the Real Culprit Please Stand Up?

Diseases and their roots are part of Satan's subtle plan to defeat us—they are part of his evil arsenal, which the Bible calls "deeds of darkness." That's why disease often works in our bodies similar to the way that sin works in the soul. It hides in the darkness of our ignorance where it can do the most damage to our health. The Bible tells us we can counter darkness by exposing it to light. Ephesians 5: 11, 13 says, "Take no part in the worthless deeds of evil and darkness; instead, rebuke and expose them...when the light shines on them, it becomes clear how evil these things are."

In the case of thyroid disorder, there generally is one underlying culprit that is the source of the illness. Interestingly, 90 percent of all thyroid disorders can be traced to this one root problem: a malfunctioning immune system, otherwise known as an *autoimmune disorder*.[1]

Our immune system was created by God to protect us against "invaders" of our bodies—such as germs and viruses—that, if left unchecked, would cause us harm and make us sick. A strong and balanced immune system will keep us in good physical health. In the case of autoimmune disorders, the immune system itself is the cause of the illness. The immune system becomes confused and mistakes healthy organs and tissues in the body for hostile invaders, attacking them and sometimes causing serious damage. Autoimmune disorders include rheumatoid arthritis, lupus, multiple sclerosis, type I diabetes, ulcerative colitis, Crohn's disease, psoriasis and scleroderma. And now we know that most thyroid disease is also caused by an autoimmune disorder.

The most common cause of *hyperthyroidism* is Graves' disease; for *hypothyroidism* the most common cause is Hashimoto's thyroiditis. Both of these diseases are autoimmune disorders in which the immune system mistakes the thyroid gland for an invader and attacks it.

Why the Confusion?

There are a number of different triggers for autoimmune disorders, some of which include pregnancy, exposure to x-rays or radiation and severe emotional stress. However, one reason your immune system gets confused may be due to our contaminated environment. (See *The Bible Cure for Autoimmune Diseases* for more information.) We come into contact with thousands of chemicals every day in our food, water and air. These man-made chemicals disrupt our hormonal balance and may be the reason for a virtual onslaught of autoimmune disorders in our country—almost at epidemic proportions.

Since the beginning of the Industrial Revolution, we have poured dangerous chemicals and pollutants into our streams, soil and air. Many are nonbiode-gradable, which means

> *One day while Jesus was teaching, some Pharisees and teachers of religious law were sitting nearby. ... And the Lord's healing power was strongly with Jesus.*
> —LUKE 5:17

they take many years to break down. That's not just in the earth, but in the human body as well! One of the main jobs of our liver is to detoxify our bodies, keeping them internally cleansed from outside pollutants. But because our bodies were never intended to cope with the hefty load of chemicals they are receiving from our polluted environment, these chemicals usually become stored within our fatty tissues. From there they may begin to confuse our immune systems. Eventually our confused immune systems may begin to attack our bodies, resulting in autoimmune diseases.

Tricking Your Body

Many of the pollutants you are exposed to every day are very similar to your body's hormones, chemically speaking. So close are they, in fact, that they can trick your body into accepting them as if they were the real thing. This is where the confusion usually begins.

These pollutants come in the form of "hormone blockers," "hormone-disrupting agents" or "hormone mimickers." Some common hormone-disrupting agents include herbicides, insecticides and fungicides.

PCBs

One well-known hormone disrupter is the *polychlorinated biphenyls*—PCBs—first introduced to the environment in 1929. PCBs were used in the electronic industry as hydraulic fluid, a lubricant and a liquid seal. They were also used in consumer products to preserve rubber, to waterproof stucco and as a basic ingredient in paint, varnish and ink. Because of their proven harmful properties, PCBs were banned in 1976. However, because of their previous widespread use, they are still rampant in our environment—beyond the reach of any government recall.[2]

Plastic containers and wraps

Plasticizers, another less well-known hormone disrupter, come from particles of plastic wrap that "migrate" into cling-wrapped food. When meat or vegetables have been wrapped in plastic in the grocery store or slices of cheese have been individually wrapped, these foods tend to absorb the plasti-

> *O LORD, you alone can heal me; you alone can save. My praises are for you alone!*
> —JEREMIAH 17:14

cizers from the wrap. When you eat this food, the plasticizers enter your body and may begin to disrupt your hormones and eventually may disrupt your immune system.

Most plastic bottles, including two-liter soda and even water bottles, contain *phthalates*, a hormone disrupter that seeps from the plastic into the soda or the water and can eventually cause health problems. It usually takes several months before the phthalates actually seep into the liquid, so it is best to buy soda or bottled water as soon after the bottling date as possible. Also, the more flexible the plastic bottle is usually indicates the more phthalates it contains. Therefore larger, thicker bottles, such as five-gallon water tanks, are safer.

Unsafe drinking water

A chemical known as *perchlorate*, which is used in rocket fuel, also has contaminated the drinking water of many different communities around the country, including Lake Mead, Nevada, and communities along the Colorado River. Perchlorate causes increased rates of hypothyroidism in newborns and can also interfere with adult thyroid function.[3]

Dental fillings

Mercury amalgams, better known as silver fillings, have been used in dentistry for over 150 years. They are actually composed of several different metals, including silver, mercury, copper and tin. The World Health Organization has estimated that the largest source of mercury in humans comes from amalgam teeth fillings—more than from all other environmental sources combined.[4] Mercury contributes to thyroid disease by binding to the thyroid gland and disrupting its function. For more information on this topic, refer to my book *What You Don't Know May Be Killing You*.

Are You a Poor Converter?

I mentioned earlier that most of the thyroid hormone in your body—about 80 percent—is called T4. T4 is important; however, another thyroid hormone is even more important. T3 is the active form of thyroid hormone (which is the hormone that actually does most of the work) and is several times stronger than T4. So, in order for your cells to get the hormone (T3)

> *Jesus traveled throughout Galilee ...[and] healed people who had every kind of sickness and disease.*
> —MATTHEW 4:23

that it needs, it must change or convert the T4 to T3.

This chemical change takes place mainly in the liver and to a less extent in the kidneys and muscles.

Many individuals whose thyroid test results are normal but who still have symptoms of hypothyroidism are simply *poor converters* of T4 to the T3 hormone. This can result from too many toxins in the liver, free-radical damage or impaired enzyme function. Below are some other lifestyle factors that can make you a poor converter or that may interfere with thyroid function.

Stress

Excessive stress can lead to adrenal fatigue, which, in turn, may lead to problems converting T4 to T3. This is especially true after your body has been through a protracted illness, a chronic injury from an accident, the stress of surgery or emotional stress. (For more information on stress, refer to *The Bible Cure for Stress*.)

Aging

As you get older, it becomes increasingly difficult for your body to keep converting T4 to T3 efficiently.

Cigarette smoking

Chronic cigarette smoking causes problems with thyroid hormone conversion.

Excessive fluoride

Fluoride has been added to most toothpaste and public drinking water to prevent cavities and tooth decay. However, too much fluoride can result in a decrease in thyroid function.

Interestingly, fluoride was once used as a medication to *slow down* an overactive thyroid!

Excessive chlorine

Chlorine is added to water—including our drinking water—to kill microorganisms. However, similar to the effect of excessive fluoride, chlorine can interfere with proper thyroid hormone conversion, and excessive intake may result in hypothyroidism.

Certain medications

Certain medications can either trigger or aggravate hypothyroidism. For example, lithium blocks the uptake of iodine, which is necessary for thyroid function, and inhibits the production and release of the thyroid hormone. Amiodarone is a medication prescribed for certain cardiac arrhythmias, but it is linked to hypothyroidism in approximately 10 percent of patients who take it.

Other medications can interfere with thyroid function, such as the antifungal drug Nizoral; antibiotics such as Bactrim and Septra; and certain diabetic drugs such as Orinase and Diabinese. Other medications, including estrogen, birth control pills, anabolic steroids and prednisone, can all affect thyroid function. Even beta blockers used to treat hypertension (such as Inderal and Tenormin) can affect thyroid function. You should always ask your physician or consult with a *Physician's Desk Reference* to determine if your medication is affecting your thyroid function.

Any of the factors named above, including being around too many toxins, may be the reason you are experiencing symptoms of low thyroid. I strongly suggest that you take immediate measures to minimize or eliminate these lifestyle factors. (For more information on this topic, read my book *Toxic Relief*.)

Stop smoking, and if you are taking synthetic hormones, discuss natural alternatives with your health provider. Minimize stress, and if you've had major surgery or experienced an injury, be sure to allow your body time to recover completely. If you are taking birth control pills and experiencing many symptoms of thyroid disease, consider asking your doctor about other methods.

Other Factors May Place You at Risk

Even if you do not smoke, have no amalgam fillings, don't take synthetic hormones and live in a relatively pollution-free environment, other factors still may be placing you at greater risk for thyroid disease.

Listed below are high-risk factors for developing hypothyroidism.

Family history

If you have a close family member—a parent, sibling, grandparent, aunt or uncle—with a thyroid disorder, your risk is higher.

Pregnancy

If you are pregnant, know that it is fairly common for women to develop postpartum hypothyroidism just after pregnancy. However, don't be alarmed. Most women's thyroid function returns to normal when the hormones associated with

> *He spoke, and they were healed—snatched from the door of death.*
> —PSALM 107:20

pregnancy and lactation also return to normal. However, hypothyroidism will continue in some women, and steps must be taken to restore thyroid function in these patients.

Exposure to radiation

Exposure to radiation, especially from receiving radioactive iodine, can increase your risk of developing hypothyroidism. Before 1970, radiation and x-ray treatments were used to treat diseases from acne to tonsillitis—even colds and adenoid problems. Today these treatments are being linked to thyroid nodules, hypothyroidism and even thyroid cancer.

Radioactive iodine has been a common treatment for Graves' disease, which in many cases leads to hypothyroidism. Thyroid surgery, such as for thyroid cancer or for large goiters, may also lead to hypothyroidism.

In Hosea 4:6, God tells us, "My people are destroyed for lack of knowledge" (NAS). But it doesn't have to be this way! God has given us the knowledge that we need to combat thyroid disorders. Even though we live in a toxic earth, we don't have to succumb to autoimmune disorders. We can start cleansing our bodies and decreasing our stress by taking steps to change our lifestyle habits. (Refer to my books *Toxic Relief, What You Don't Know May Be Killing You* and *The Bible Cure for Autoimmune Diseases* for information on these topics.)

Live in the Light

As you continue to read through this Bible Cure book, the Lord is lighting a path of understanding for you so that no hidden problem can rob you of your health. The psalmist wrote, "LORD, you have brought light to my life; my God, you light up my darkness" (Ps. 18:28). Allow Him, and He will light a pathway into His own healing, restoring, cleansing presence that you've never before imagined was possible. He invites you to walk in the light of His wonderful love.

> *Have compassion on me, LORD, for I am weak.*
> —PSALM 6:2

If you long to know Him better, if you seek His healing touch, ask Him now, "Lord, let me live in the light of Your truth." If you think you may have a thyroid condition that is due to an underlying autoimmune disorder, pray the following prayer with me right now.

A Bible Cure Prayer
FOR YOU

Heavenly Father, You created my body to function in perfect harmony, and my immune system was intended to protect me from any outside invaders that would cause me harm. God, it is not Your will that my immune system is confused and attacking my thyroid gland, and that it is an unhealthy invader. I thank You for restoring order and peace within my body right now and that all of my bodily systems line up with Your Word. In Jesus' name, amen.

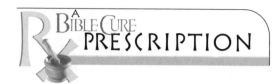

Take an inventory of the disruptive agents to which you are exposed in your daily lifestyle.

- ❑ What sources of plastic pollution do you encounter daily?

- ❑ Is your mouth filled with silver (mercury) fillings?

- ❑ What other disruptive agents and medications do you feel may be affecting your health?

- ❑ Are you willing to trust God to help you change your lifestyle and lessen your health risk from environmental contaminants?

Chapter 3

Brighter and Brighter— Supplements

Many believe that God's teachings are for our mind and spirit only. Yet, God created our entire being—body, mind and spirit. If we allow Him, He will teach us wisdom to light a pathway of healing and understanding. The Bible says, "For these commands and this teaching are a lamp to light the way ahead of you" (Prov. 6:23).

God is determined to stop your enemies of sickness and disease from keeping you from His perfect plan for your life. Psalm 30:1–2 says, "You refused to let my enemies triumph over me. O LORD my God, I cried out to you for help, and you restored my health."

No matter how dark your circumstances or physical symptoms may seem at the moment, when you look to God for help they get brighter and brighter. "The way of the righteous is like the first gleam of dawn, which shines ever brighter until the full light of day" (Prov. 4:18).

So, be encouraged, and get ready to start feeling much better, for there is much you can do to turn your situation completely around. You have already seen how lifestyle factors can make a great difference in how your thyroid functions. Let's shine the light a little brighter by taking a look at some natural substances God has placed in His great creation that can help you gain victory.

Necessary Nutrients for a Healthy Thyroid

Iodine

Iodine, from seawater, is a natural substance found in abundance throughout the earth. As we've seen, getting too little or too much iodine can dramatically impact thyroid health. Too much can lead to hyperthyroidism and can actually trigger the autoimmune response, and too little can lead to goiters and other thyroid problems. Low iodine levels are actually a leading cause of thyroid dysfunction in the world at large, although it is not as great a factor in developed countries such the U.S. and European countries where table salt is iodized.

Yet, many Americans who have banned all salt from their diets for health reasons are starting to experience problems. More and more bakeries and restaurants also feature low-salt or no-salt selections. A study in the *Journal of Clinical Endocrinology and Metabolism* in October of 1998 showed that the iodine levels measured in urine excretion had fallen by half compared to tests of earlier studies done for people living in the U.S. It cited that 12 percent of Americans had low iodine concentrations in their urine compared to

> *Dear friend, I am praying that all is well with you and that your body is as healthy as I know your soul is.*
> —3 John 2

1994, when less than 1 percent of the population had low levels of iodine.[1]

The American Heart Association recommends that we get a teaspoon of salt every day (6 grams, which contains approximately 400 mcg of iodine).[2]

Since nature's primary source of iodine is seawater, the closer you live to the sea the better off you are, at least in respect to getting enough iodine in your body. If you live in the central plains or near the Great Lakes, then your body is dependent upon the iodine you receive in your table salt and food that comes from the sea.

If you are on a low-salt diet and rarely eat ocean fish and seafood, onions or dairy products, I recommend taking a daily multivitamin/multimineral supplement that contains 150 mcg of iodine. Use iodized salt or, even better, use sea salt or Celtic salt. The RDA for adults is 150 mcg a day, and, fortunately, the usual daily intake in the U.S. is about 150 to 550 mcg per day.

> *The sick begged [Jesus] to let them at least touch the fringe of his robe, and all who touched it were healed.*
> —MARK 6:56

Caution: Balance is very important where iodine is involved, for we've seen that it can be a double-edged sword. Too much or too little iodine can lead to thyroid problems. Therefore, do not take large doses of kelp or other supplements high in iodine since they may trigger hyperthyroidism.

Tyrosine

The thyroid gland actually needs two different nutrients from the diet: the first is iodine, and the second is *tyrosine*. Tyrosine is an amino acid that the body forms from the metabolism of the essential amino acid *phenylalanine*. In fact, the body makes most of the tyrosine it needs from phenylalanine, so tyrosine is not considered an essential amino acid to add to the diet, although it is helpful to do so.

Foods that are high in tyrosine include chicken, fish, soybeans, bananas, dairy foods, almonds and lima beans. Be sure to include plenty of these items in your regular diet in order to get enough tyrosine.

Let's take a look at some supplements that will give good results.

Super Supplements

If you have a thyroid disorder, or a borderline thyroid disorder, supplements can help bring your body back into the right balance. Here are some supplements you may take.

A good multivitamin/multimineral

Your multivitamin should contain vitamin A, vitamin B_2, B_6, B_{12}, vitamin C and zinc. Moderate amounts of these substances are essential for making thyroid hormone. Zinc is essential, but it must also be balanced with copper in a 10:1 ratio. It's unwise to economize when it comes to vitamins, since quality varies widely among brands. The best brands generally will yield the best results. Divine Health Multivitamins is a high-quality brand. You can order it from my Web site at www.drcolbert.com.

Selenium

Selenium, an important antioxidant, is one of the most important nutrients your body uses to convert thyroid hormone to meet your body's needs. Interestingly, Brazil nuts contain a whopping 840 mcg of selenium per ounce—twelve times as much as you need each day.

The RDA for selenium is 70 mcg, so check your label as dosages can vary widely from brand to brand.

Dosage: Take a multivitamin that contains at least 100 mcg of selenium, or take a selenium supplement. You may choose to simply eat a Brazil nut a day.

Moducare and Natur-Leaf

Moducare and Natur-Leaf are blends of plant sterols and sterolins that work to restore, strengthen and balance your body's immune system. Plant sterols and sterolins are natural substances found in all fruits, vegetables, nuts and seeds.

Because they help to balance the immune system, Moducare or Natur-Leaf may prove effective in helping treat both Hashimoto's thyroiditis, the leading cause of hypothyroidism, and Graves' disease, the leading cause of hyperthyroidism.

Plant sterols and sterolins generally also have an anti-inflammatory effect. They also may be able to modulate the autoimmune response. I recommend plant sterols and sterolins especially for patients with Graves' disease.

Moducare, which can be found at most health food stores, is one of the most popular of the plant sterol treatments. Natur-Leaf may be ordered by calling 1-800-532-7845.

Dosage for Moducare: Adults can take one capsule three times daily, or two capsules upon rising and one at bedtime. This dose may need to be increased to two to three

> *O Lord my God,*
> *I cried out to*
> *you for help, and*
> *you restored my*
> *health.*
> —Psalm 30:2

capsules three times per day, taken one hour before meals. The dose for Natur-Lear is generally one capsule two times a day one hour before meals, but it may need to be increased to two capsules two times a day. Since Moducare and Natur-Leaf are similar products, I recommend that you take one or the other.

A Marvelous Symphony

Do you remember the old children's song "Dry Bones"? The song went on and on about each part of the body being connected to the other parts of the body.

The incredible intricacy and complexity of the human body can never be fully expressed in a children's song. That's because your body's complex systems work together like a marvelous symphony orchestrated to perfection, with each part vitally connected to the others, working together to keep you healthy and happy.

The endocrine system, which is made up of the various glands in your body, is a vital part of that grand symphony. Each gland is interconnected and communicates with all of the other glands. The hypothalamus, pituitary gland, thyroid gland, adrenal glands and reproductive glands all work closely together. When there is an imbalance in one gland, such as the adrenal glands or the reproductive glands, it can, in turn, put a strain on the functioning of the thyroid gland.

Stressed Out Adrenals?

Your adrenal glands produce many different hormones, including cortisol, DHEA, progesterone, pregnenolone, testosterone and estrogen. When you are under a lot of stress for a prolonged period of time, these vitally important glands can begin producing excessive cortisol. Excessive cortisol production may eventually lead to adrenal fatigue and possibly adrenal exhaustion accompanied by low cortisol production. Both of these states—excessive cortisol production and low cortisol production—can make you a poor converter of T4 to T3. Remember, T3 is the active form of thyroid hormone and is several times stronger than T4.

DSF

During extended times of stress, you can help your body to balance its production of cortisol by supplementing with DSF. This de-stress formula is carefully blended to help restore the body's adrenal function. You can purchase this excellent supplement from Nutri-West by calling 1-800-451-5620.

Dosage: Take at least one chewable tablet twice a day at breakfast and lunch.

DHEA

DHEA is a hormone made naturally by your adrenal glands. Many call it the "youth" hormone because low levels are linked to aging. When your adrenals are exhausted, often your supply of

DHEA is low, which causes hormonal regulation in your entire body to suffer. When your cortisol levels are high, DHEA levels are usually low. You can replenish this vital hormone by taking it in supplement form.

Dosage: Take a small amount of DHEA under the tongue once a day (women 5 mg a day; men, 10 mg a day).

For more information on the adrenal glands, please refer to *The Bible Cure for Stress*. To order DHEA, visit our Web site at www.drcolbert.com.

A BIBLE CURE HEALTH TIP

Screen Your Own Adrenals

You can screen yourself to find out if your adrenal glands are functioning optimally. Here's how.

THE BLOOD PRESSURE TEST

Take your own blood pressure while lying down after you've been at rest for a moderate length of time. Record your reading in the space below.

_____

Stand up and immediately take your blood pressure again. Write it in the space below.

_____

Evaluation: (check one)

❏ My blood pressure stayed the same.

❏ My blood pressure rose.

❏ My blood pressure dropped.

If your blood pressure went up or stayed the same, your adrenals are probably in fairly good shape. However, if your blood pressure dropped after you stood up, there is a good chance you are suffering from adrenal fatigue.[3]

If you are not equipped to accurately read your own blood pressure, try this test instead. You will need the help of a close friend.

THE PUPIL DILATION TEST: ROGOFF'S SIGN

In a dark room, have a close friend shine a flashlight directly into your eye for approximately thirty seconds. He or she will be evaluating the size of your pupil. Your pupil will need to be watched very closely.

Normal pupil: If your pupil is normal it will constrict in the light and remain small.

Abnormal pupil: If your pupil wavers, dilates or does not constrict, it is abnormal. Any of these abnormal reactions suggest your body is experiencing adrenal fatigue.

Check It Out

I strongly suggest that you have all of your hormone levels checked and that you begin supplementing any hormones you are lacking. Both those with hypothyroidism and hyperthyroidism generally have low adrenal reserves and would benefit greatly from DHEA and DSF.

Natural testosterone or progesterone

One final note: Because of the close association between the various glands—including the reproductive glands—I have found that many people with thyroid disorders have low levels of sex hormones.

If you have a thyroid disorder, you may need to have your sex hormones checked. Women may need phytoestrogens and a natural progesterone cream, along with small amounts of natural testosterone cream. Salivary hormone testing of adrenal hormones and sex hormones is a simple test to screen for imbalances of these hormones.

Take Warning

You may be especially health conscious and currently take several supplements in order to strengthen your body. But if you have a thyroid disorder, you may need to reexamine what you're taking. Some supplements may actually aggravate your condition.

Lipoic acid

Lipoic acid is a powerful antioxidant used by many physicians to treat diabetes, hepatitis and psoriasis. However, lipoic acid may make you a poor converter, decreasing your ability to convert T4 to T3. That's the reason that some people who take lipoic acid begin exhibiting many of the symptoms of hypothyroidism.

If you have begun to take lipoic acid and have developed several symptoms of a low thyroid, you may need to either lower your dose or stop taking it altogether.

Kelp and bladderwrack

These herbs are known for having many health benefits, but they also contain lots of iodine. And as you've seen, too much iodine can increase your risk for developing hyperthyroidism. That's especially true if you are getting plenty of iodine in your table salt.

If you have symptoms of thyroid disorder and are taking either of these herbs, I encourage you to find other supplements containing less iodine.

Treating Hypothyroidism

Synthetic (man-made) preparations

If you have hypothyroidism, no supplement or herb can substitute for what you really need, which is thyroid hormone. Your physician will probably start you on T4, which is supplied by the major synthetic brands of T4 thyroid hormones (Synthroid, Levothroid, Levoxyl and Unithroid). Some patients, for whatever reason, don't respond as well to generic synthetic T4 hormone preparations, and so I recommend that you take the major brands mentioned above.

> *Don't be afraid, for I am with you. Do not be dismayed, for I am your God. I will strengthen you. I will help you. I will uphold you with my victorious right hand.*
> —ISAIAH 41:10

Synthetic T4 thyroid hormones are the standard treatment of choice for most doctors. Very rarely will a medical doctor stray from prescribing one of the four preparations listed above, or a generic version of them. *Synthroid* remains the top-selling thyroid hormone in the United States—its generic substitute is called *levothyroxine*.

As you have learned, many patients are unable to successfully convert the T4 hormone to T3, yet their thyroid tests are normal. For these patients, the synthetic T3 hormone called *liothyronine* may be effective. Its product name is *Cytomel*. A small amount of Cytomel in a sustained-released preparation will often relieve the symptoms of hypothyroidism in these individuals. These sustained released preparations of thyroid hormone can only be obtained from a compounding pharmacy such as Pharmacy Specialists. Your physician can contact them at 1-407-260-7002.

Most physicians, however, only prescribe the T4 hormone such as Synthroid. I believe that in the future, more doctors will begin to provide an appropriate mixture of T4 and T3, which is more similar to the actual hormone secretion of the thyroid gland.

A More Natural Path

Perhaps you've determined that you prefer to treat your hypothyroidism condition with more natural methods. Staying as close to nature as possible is often best. Nevertheless, you may imagine that only those with borderline thyroid disease have that option. But you're wrong. Natural medications exist even for those with long-term hypothyroidism. Let's take a look at some more natural options.

Natural thyroid hormone preparations, including Armour Thyroid, Biotech Thyroid, Westhroid and Naturethroid, are medications produced from the desiccated thyroid glands of pigs. They contain both T4 and T3 hormones. Each of these natural thyroid products is essentially the same—they just have different fillers. One important note: If you have allergies to corn, take the Biotech or Naturethroid products, which have no corn fillers.

With my own patients, I generally prescribe a natural thyroid hormone such as those listed above.

Again, many individuals with hypothyroidism take some form of synthetic T4, usually Synthroid, but may not be getting all the T3 they need, since many are poor converters of T4 to T3. This is the reason why they may continue

> *Yes, your healing will come quickly. Your godliness will lead you forward, and the glory of the LORD will protect you from behind.*
> —ISAIAH 58:8

to exhibit symptoms of hypothyroidism. By switching to a natural thyroid hormone or simply by adding a small amount of sustained-release T3, most symptoms of hypothyroidism can be eliminated.

A BIBLE CURE HEALTHTIP

Tips for Taking Thyroid Hormone Supplements

❑ Take thyroid hormone mediations about the same time each day.

❑ Don't take thyroid medication with other medications.

❑ It is critically important to take the thyroid hormone on an empty stomach with water so that it can be absorbed efficiently.

❑ Do not take thyroid hormones with iron supplements—wait at least two to three hours after taking the thyroid hormone before taking an iron supplement.

❑ Wait at least three to four hours after taking a thyroid supplement before taking any calcium. This includes milk and even orange juice, since most orange juice has been fortified with calcium.

❑ Take multivitamins, which generally contain both iron and calcium, at least three hours after taking the thyroid hormone.

❑ Do not take antacids, such as Maalox or Mylanta, with the thyroid hormone. Wait at least two to three hours after taking a thyroid hormone before taking these medications.

Gaining Against Graves'

The standard medical treatment for Graves' disease, which is hyperthyroidism, has benefits and also a downside. Let's take a look.

Radioactive iodine

The most common treatment for Graves' disease is radioactive iodine 131 (RAI). This treatment actually destroys cells in the thyroid gland so that it becomes unable to produce thyroid hormone. Unfortunately, many patients who undergo this treatment go to the other extreme and develop hypothyroidism.

Antithyroid medication

For my patients with Graves' disease, I prefer to prescribe antithyroid medication, particularly methimazole or Tapazole. This medication blocks the production of thyroid hormone without destroying the cells of the thyroid gland itself.

Armed With Understanding

The next time you see your doctor, you will go armed with a greater understanding about your thyroid condition. Realize too that, with the power of the knowledge you have gained in this book, you now have more than one choice of medication. Most doctors will simply prescribe Synthroid (synthetic T4), but you've gained the option of finding a physician who can prescribe a natural thyroid medication, such as Armour Thyroid, Naturethroid or Biotech Thyroid. Even if you cannot find such a doctor, your own doctor might be willing to add T3 hormone to your regimen.

> *He comforts us in all our troubles so that we can comfort others. When others are troubled, we will be able to give them the same comfort God has given us.*
> —2 CORINTHIANS 1:4

55

A Great Physician

Wisdom and knowledge alone are not enough in themselves. As you seek healing for your condition, always seek the Healer first. All healing comes from Him.

Often His healing power comes into your life as a rising light that shines with greater and greater power as it flows into you and through you to everyone you meet. The Bible says, "The Sun of Righteousness will rise with healing in his wings" (Mal. 4:2). I believe this brightness of His rising is already beginning to shine upon your life.

Fortunately, we have the Great Physician on our side, the One who possesses all the keys to knowledge and wisdom and who loves us with an everlasting love. Turn to Him and begin to seek His wisdom and healing power.

A BIBLE CURE PRAYER
FOR YOU

Dear heavenly Father, I know that You are the Creator of the universe and the Creator of my body. I thank You that You understand the mysterious intricacies that make up the systems of my body and that it is Your will that they all function together in perfect harmony. Lord, I place my thyroid gland and all of its functions into Your capable hands. You are the Healer, the Great Physician, and I trust You with my condition. Teach me the things that I need to do, the areas I may need to change, in order to walk in Your divine health. And give me the grace and the discipline I need to follow through. In Jesus' name, amen.

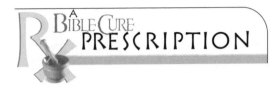

List the supplements you are planning to speak with your physician about taking.

_____

_____

_____

What sources of iodine are you getting in your diet?

_____

_____

_____

Based upon the information you read in this chapter, should you make any changes to your iodine intake? If so, what are they?

_____

_____

_____

What good multivitamin/multimineral supplement are you taking at present?

_____

_____

_____

What sources of selenium are you presently getting in your diet?

_____

_____

_____

Do you believe you may be a poor converter of T4 to T3? Why?

_____

_____

_____

Chapter 4

A Lighted Temple—Nutrition

Walking in the light of God's wisdom will actually change your physical appearance. The Bible says, "How wonderful to be wise, to be able to analyze and interpret things. Wisdom lights up a person's face, softening its hardness" (Eccles. 8:1).

In fact, your entire being can shine in the light of God's truth. The Book of Daniel says, "Those who are wise will shine like the brightness of the heavens, and those who lead many to righteousness, like the stars for ever and ever" (Dan. 12:3, NIV).

Daniel was a wise young man who had a spirit of excellence. Interestingly, one of the ways he displayed excellence that pleased God greatly was through his dietary choices. For when the banquets of kings were placed before him, menus that were doubtless filled with fatty meats, sugary sweets and the most refined breads and cakes available in the kingdom, Daniel refused to indulge. Even at the risk of punishment, he chose to eat only vegetables.

Why? He wisely understood that his food choices made a great difference in both the natural and spiritual realms. This excellent young man realized his body was a temple of the Holy Spirit, and he refused to eat anything that might defile it.

America's Rich Man's Diet

Proverbs 23:1–3 says, "When dining with a ruler, pay attention to what is put before you. If you are a big eater, put a knife to your throat, and don't desire all the delicacies—deception may be involved." Here the Bible warns us against the "deception" of eating what is pleasing to our palates but may not nourish and strengthen our bodies. In fact, much of the rich, sugary, refined foods historically eaten by the rich were genuinely bad for the body. The simpler whole-grain breads, fish and vegetables of peasants who lived closer to the natural earth were far healthier.

Amazingly, America's "rich man's diet" of excessive sweets and refined, processed foods and fatty meats has created an epidemic of sickness. It is estimated that 75 percent of all deaths each year are related to inadequate nutrition.[1] It's no wonder that God gave such a strong warning against the "deceptive food" of refined, processed and sugary items that taste good but do not adequately nourish the body.

Your body is the temple of God. First Corinthians 6:19 says, "Or don't you know that your body is the temple of the Holy Spirit, who lives in you and was given to you by God? You do not belong to yourself." What you put into your temple will determine a great deal about your health—both physically and spiritually. Daniel refused to defile his temple. What about you?

If you have thyroid disease or its symptoms, you may need to reject certain dietary choices in order to protect and heal your body. You have an excellent spirit just like Daniel, and with God's help you can begin implementing this Bible cure step of making good nutritional choices. As God shines His wonderful Spirit upon you, your temple will be increasingly filled with His glorious light.

> *Don't be impressed with your own wisdom. Instead, fear the LORD and turn your back on evil. Then you will gain renewed health and vitality.*
> —PROVERBS 3:7–8

Let's turn now and explore this vital Bible cure step.

You Are What You Eat

An old expression says, "You are what you eat." In other words, eating good, healthy foods will give your body strong, powerful nutrients with which to build and repair itself. Providing your body with inferior nutrition can make it weak and easily susceptible to infirmity and disease.

Begin this Bible cure step by determining to rid your diet of selections that weaken your immune system and undermine your overall balance of health.

Reject

Reject all highly processed foods, refined grains, starches and sugars.

Prefer

Eat plenty of fresh vegetables, fresh fruits and unrefined, complex carbohydrates. Here's a good rule of thumb: The closer to the garden you eat, the better. The farther away from the garden—in terms of processing and refining—the worse off your food selections will be.

Go Organic

Organic foods are becoming increasingly popular and easier to find. Many food chains now carry organic varieties of just about everything. The prices for organic foods are going down, too. Although organics may still cost a little more, the health benefits are well worth it. Here's why.

Fruits and vegetables

Organic fruits and vegetables will decrease your exposure to hormone-disruptive substances. These include the pesticides, synthetic hormones and other toxins we discussed in chapter one. Therefore, as often as you can, choose organically grown vegetables and fruits. When you cannot, be aggressive in carefully washing your fruits and vegetables with warm water and a mild soap, or try using one of the popular vegetable cleansing products available at health food stores. Be sure to rinse well after washing.

Dairy products

Choose organic milk, eggs and dairy products. Non-organic varieties may contain hormones and antibiotics, both of which can dramatically impact your thyroid function. Also choose low-fat or nonfat dairy products.

Meats

Free-range meats are not fed hormones and other drugs to fatten them up. If you can afford it, choose these whenever possible. When purchasing non-free-range meats, select the leanest cuts and carefully trim off the fat and skin. Hormone-disrupting chemicals are primarily concentrated in the fat of the animal, so significantly reducing the amount of animal fat in your diet will make a big difference.

Danger: NutraSweet Can Harm You!

Do you drink iced tea throughout the day and add that little blue packet of sweetener? Or do you enjoy a diet soda in the afternoons? If so, the aspartame in these products could be affecting your thyroid.

Researchers are discovering that aspartame can have a dramatic negative impact on the thyroid.[2] If you have hypothyroidism, Graves' disease or Hashimoto's thyroiditis, or if you have symptoms indicating you may be developing either of these thyroid diseases, I strongly encourage you avoid using all products that contain aspartame, or NutraSweet.

Opposite Ends of the Spectrum

Because *hypothyroidism* (too little thyroid hormone) and *hyperthyroidism* (too much thyroid hormone) are opposite ends of the delicate thyroid hormone balance, those with either of these conditions will at times receive vastly different advice. Consider these thyroid disorders as book ends.

Check out the specific dietary advice concerning your particular situation very carefully. Don't be surprised to discover that you may need to do exactly the opposite of what someone at the other end of the balance scale needs to do.

Soy Products and Your Thyroid

Normally I encourage my patients to eat soy products, as long as they are not allergic to them. However, eating a lot of soy products is unwise if you are struggling to overcome an underactive thyroid, or *hypothyroidism*. Soy products suppress thyroid function.

Soy products—including soybeans, soy milk and soy protein—contain isoflavins. Isoflavins, such as *genistein,* block iodine and tyrosine, preventing them from producing the thyroid hormone. In addition, check to determine whether other supplements you are taking contain genistein or other isoflavins. If so, decrease or avoid these products that tend to suppress thyroid function further.

For those with an underactive thyroid, soy products can promote the formation of goiters as well as trigger autoimmune thyroid disease.

Now, if you have *hyperthyroidism*, or an overactive thyroid, soy products will usually prove beneficial to you, since your body is producing too much thyroid hormone and soy products tend to slow that process down.

Don't Eat These With Hypothyroidism

Certain foods are called *goitrogens* because eating them in excessive amounts can lead to the formation of goiters and hypothyroidism (an underactive thyroid). This is caused by cyanide derivatives contained in the plants. Because cooking them thoroughly usually inactivates the goitrogens, if you have low thyroid function, limit the amount of foods you consume raw; instead, steam or cook them.

Goitrogen foods primarily consist of raw vegetables, especially cruciferous ones. These include:

- Broccoli
- Cabbage
- Cauliflower
- Brussels sprouts

- Kale
- Turnip and mustard greens

Besides these vegetables, other goitrogens include:

- Sweet corn
- Millet
- Pine nuts
- Peanuts
- Almonds
- Walnuts

When these foods make up a major part of your diet, especially if eaten raw, they can create a risk factor for hypothyroidism. However, I'm not suggesting that you cut out these foods completely from your diet. Merely limit them, and steam or cook cruciferous vegetables before eating them.

Do Eat These With Hyperthyroidism

Conversely, if you have *hyperthyroidism*, certain foods that those with *hypothyroidism* must limit are actually good for you. While these foods are not good for patients who have an underactive thyroid gland, they have beneficial effects for an overactive thyroid. They can slow down a hyper-active thyroid, much like pressing on the brakes of a car. You may eat plenty of the following:

- Broccoli
- Cauliflower
- Cabbage
- Brussels sprouts
- Sweet corn
- Millet
- Peanuts
- Almonds
- Walnuts

Don't Eat These With Hyperthyroidism

Because excessive iodine intake helps promote hyperthyroidism, too much of it in your diet can intensify symptoms of hyperthyroidism when you are battling Graves' disease. Therefore, if your thyroid is overactive, limit these selections:

- Ocean fish
- Shellfish
- Dairy products
- Kelp and other forms of seaweed
- Onions
- Asparagus

All of these selections are loaded with iodine. In addition, many bakeries add extra salt and iodine to dough to make it easier to work with. In fact, a slice of bread typically contains about 150 mcg of iodine. This is another powerful reason to limit your intake of processed foods.

Fatten Up

Another symptom of Graves' disease (an overactive thyroid) is weight loss, especially muscle mass. If you are battling hyperthyroidism, you are probably prone to losing too much muscle weight. Therefore, you need to eat a diet high in protein to counteract the muscle loss you are experiencing. I also recommend 100 mcg a day of coenzyme Q_{10} to protect the heart, which is a muscle.

Consume even more calories than usual—especially unrefined, complex carbohydrates, proteins and "good" fats. Eat often, every three to four hours, to prevent weight loss.

The Wonder of Water

To combat any thyroid condition, it is extremely important to drink adequate amounts of water—at least two quarts day.

Also, stop drinking tap water; drink filtered water instead. Reverse-osmosis-filtered water is some of the cleanest water you can drink, and it generally doesn't contain hormone-disrupting chemicals, fluoride, chlorine or other chemicals, which can affect the thyroid.

If you decide to drink bottled water, make sure that you know the date that the water was bottled, and drink it as close to that date as possible—at least within a month or two—in order to decrease your exposure to plasticizers or phthalates.

A BIBLE CURE HEALTH TIP

How Much Water Do I Need?

Here's a good way to find out how much water you really need to drink every day.

Write down your weight in pounds _____

Divide that number by 2 _____

Remainder = _____

The remainder is the number of ounces of water you need to drink daily.

Be a Doer

The Bible encourages us, "Be ye doers of the word, and not hearers only" (James 1:22, KJV). This is good advice, even as it applies to practical nutritional wisdom for good health. By learning about and implementing these simple health strategies, you are now armed with the knowledge you need to combat your thyroid disorder. Knowledge is power, and when put into use, it becomes wisdom for prevention and healing for yourself and others.

A BIBLE CURE PRAYER
FOR YOU

Lord Jesus, thank You so much for the knowledge and wisdom You have provided in this book. I ask You for Your help and guidance as I begin to implement these strategies in my life. Continue to further the healing that You have begun in my body as I learn to walk in Your ways. Thank You for Your healing power that is always available to me. As I go forth in health and wholeness, I will share Your love and mercy with others and begin to follow the plan that You have designed for my life. In Jesus' name I pray all of these things, amen.

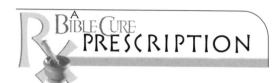

Write your particular thyroid condition in the space below.

_____

_____

_____

What foods will you eat to help with your healing?

_____

_____

_____

What foods will you reject?

_____

_____

_____

How much water do you drink per day?

_____

_____

_____

How much should you be drinking according to the Health Tip in this chapter?

_____

_____

Write out a strategy to help you drink more water every day.

_____

_____

Record your commitment to God to be a doer and not a hearer only.

_____

_____

_____

_____

_____

_____

_____

_____

Chapter 5

Arise, Shine—Faith

When your body is bright with a radiant glow of vibrant health, your light will shine to others all around you. The Bible says, "Then Jesus asked them, 'Would anyone light a lamp and then put it under a basket or under a bed to shut out the light? Of course not! A lamp is placed on a stand, where its light will shine'" (Mark 4:21).

This book would be incomplete without the final Bible cure step: faith. In order to walk in the radiant glow of health that God intends for you, you must step out in faith and boldly receive His very best.

What Is Faith?

Faith is not a dove or a cloud. It's not a gift that some have and others lack. It's not an eerie force, and it's not the "luck of the draw" or what happens to those who win the lottery.

Faith is choosing to believe God, no matter

what anyone else says, no matter what your eyes see or your ears hear. Faith determines to choose to believe that God is your healer, that He loves you and that He desires to see you well.

Right now you have all the faith you need to experience a total healing in your body. The Bible says all it takes is a little, tiny kernel of faith, no bigger than a mustard seed.

Faith simply takes God at His Word. That's why faith is simple enough for a child to grasp.

Rise and Shine

The Book of Isaiah commands, "Arise, shine; for your light has come, and the glory of the LORD has risen upon you" (Isa. 60:1, NAS). Faith always demands action. You must be the one who determines to arise. When you do so, you can be sure that you will shine because the glorious light of God's presence will rise upon your life.

Why not choose to rise up in faith and claim God's promises this very moment? If bold, unwavering faith is your choice right now, then step out on God's promise by bowing your head and praying this prayer. Get ready to let your light shine brightly!

A BIBLE CURE PRAYER
FOR YOU

Lord Jesus, You are the amazing Healer. You hold the keys to all power, wisdom and understanding—the very earth itself was created by Your will and Your hand. But I know that You are also my Savior—that You bore the stripes on Your back so that my healing could take place. Lord, I trust You with my condition. I believe that You have the power to heal me, and not only that, You want to heal me! I place myself in Your hands and ask that Your healing power would flow in me and through me. Let the healing of my condition take place and be a witness and a testimony to Your power and love. I declare today that I choose faith. I receive Your healing power right now. In Jesus' name, amen.

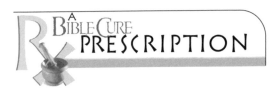

Faith Builder

He was pierced through for our transgressions, He was crushed for our iniquities; the chastening for our well-being
fell upon Him, and by His scourging we
are healed.

—Isaiah 53:5, NAS

Read this dynamic scripture aloud several times. It has great power! Insert your own name into it.

He was pierced through for _____ transgressions, He was crushed for _____ iniquities; the chastening of _____ well-being fell upon Him, and by His scourging _____ _____ is healed!

Now write a prayer thanking God for your healing.

_____

_____

_____

A PERSONAL NOTE

From Don and Mary Colbert

God desires to heal you of disease. His Word is full of promises that confirm His love for you and His desire to give you His abundant life. His desire includes more than physical health for you; He wants to make you whole in your mind and spirit as well through a personal relationship with His Son, Jesus Christ.

If you haven't met our best friend, Jesus, we would like to take this opportunity to introduce Him to you. It is very simple.

If you are ready to let Him come into your heart and become your best friend, just bow your head and sincerely pray this prayer from your heart:

> *Lord Jesus, I want to know You as my Savior and Lord. I believe You are the Son of God and that You died for my sins. I also believe You were raised from the dead and now sit at the right hand of the Father praying for me. I ask You to forgive me for my sins and change my heart so that I can be Your child and live with*

You eternally. Thank You for Your peace.
Help me to walk with You so that I can
begin to know You as my best friend and
my Lord. Amen.

If you have prayed this prayer, we rejoice with you in your decision and your new relationship with Jesus. Please contact us at pray4me@strang.com so that we can send you some materials that will help you become established in your relationship with the Lord. You have just made the most important decision of your life. We look forward to hearing from you.

Notes

PREFACE

1. L. A. McKeown, "Everyone Over 35 Needs Thyroid Test, Group Says," WebMD Health, http://my.webmd.com/content/article/26/1728_58533.htm (accessed November 23, 2003).

2. Richard Shames, M.D., and Karilee H. Shames, Ph.D., *Thyroid Power: Ten Steps to Total Health* (New York: HarperCollins, 2001), 2.

CHAPTER 1

1. Mary Shoman, "Breaking News: Estrogen, Menopause and Thyroid," http://thyroid.about.com/library/weekly/aa042602a.htm (accessed November 23, 2003).

2. P. W. Ladenson, et al., "American Thyroid Association's Guidelines for Detection of Thyroid Dysfunction," *Arch Intern Med.* 160 (2000): 1573–1575.

3. Elizabeth Smoots, M.D., FAAFP, "Is My Thyroid Overactive?", WebMD Health, http://my.webmd.com/content/article/42/1689_50865.htm? (accessed November 23, 2003).

4. The National Women's Health Information Center, "Graves' Disease," October 23, 2000, http://www.4woman.gov/faq/graves.htm (accessed November 23, 2003).

5. M. Sara Rosenthal, *The Thyroid Sourcebook* (Los Angeles: Lowell, 2000).

6. Ibid.

CHAPTER 2

1. Glen Rothfeld, *Thyroid Balance* (Avon, MA: Adams Media, 2003).

2. Theo Colborn, et al., *Our Stolen Future* (New York: Plume Books, 1997), ii.

3. For more information on this topic, see www.perchlorateinfo.com.

4. David Kennedy, *Health Consciousness* 13 (3): 92–93.

CHAPTER 3

1. Joseph G. Hollowell, et al., "Iodine Nutrition in the United States. Trends and Public Health Implications: Iodine Excretion Data from National Health and Nutrition Examination Surveys I and III," *Journal of Clinical Endocrinology and Metabolism* 83 (10) (1998): 3401–3408.

2. For more information, see www.heartcenteronline.com.

3. Gonzzo Watson, D.C., "Adrenal Fatigue and a Holistic Approach to Recovery," http://www.watsonchiropractic.com/articles/adftg.htm (accessed November 24, 2003).

CHAPTER 4

1. "Fighting Death, Disease, and Discomfort," NutritionStreet.com; http://www.nutitionstreet.com/fightingdisease.shtml: "The former Surgeon General of the United States, C. Everett Koop said of the 2.1 million deaths each year, 1.6 million (or 75 percent) were related to inadequate diet."

2. H. Roberts, *Aspartame Disease: An Ignored Epidemic* (N.p.: Sunshine Sentinel Press, 2001), 432.

DON COLBERT, M.D., was born in Tupelo, Mississippi. He attended Oral Roberts University School of Medicine in Tulsa, Oklahoma, where he received a bachelor of science degree in biology in addition to his degree in medicine. Dr. Colbert completed his internship and residency with Florida Hospital in Orlando, Florida. He is board certified in family practice and has received extensive training in nutritional medicine.

If you would like more
information about natural and
divine healing, or information about
Divine Health Nutritional Products,
you may contact Dr. Colbert at:

DR. DON COLBERT
1908 Boothe Circle
Longwood, FL 32750
Telephone: 407–331–7007
(For ordering products only)
Dr. Colbert's Web site is
www.drcolbert.com.

Disclaimer: Dr. Colbert and the staff of Divine Health Wellness Center are prohibited from addressing a patient's medical condition by phone, facsimile or e-mail. Please refer questions related to your medical condition to your own primary care physician.